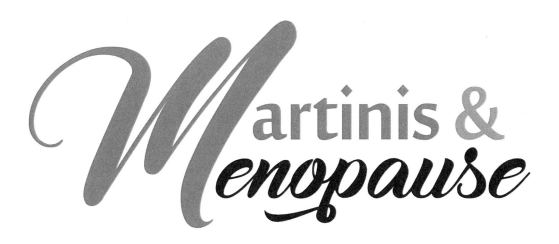

Martinis & Menopause

A Companion
Workbook

This workbook is a conversation starter–
a companion, guide, and resource for your journey through menopause.
Enjoy!

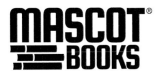

www.mascotbooks.com

Martinis and Menopause
A Companion Workbook

This book is not intended as a substitute for the medical advice of physicians. The reader should regularly consult a physician in matters relating to his/her health and particularly with respect to any symptoms that may require diagnosis or medical attention.

For more information, please contact:

Mascot Books

620 Herndon Parkway, Suite 320

Herndon, VA 20170

info@mascotbooks.com

CPSIA Code: PRR0619A

ISBN-13: 978-1-64307-455-9

Printed in the United States

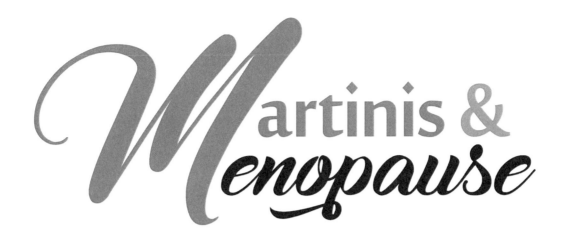

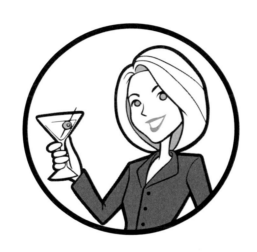

A Companion
Workbook

Kelli Jaecks

Table of Contents

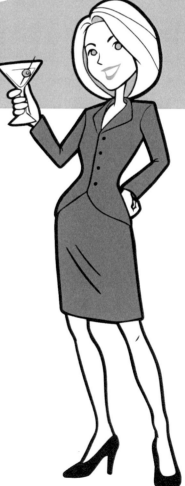

Introduction

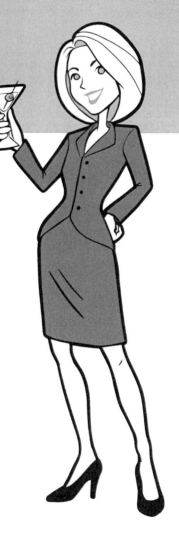

As Heraclitus said,
"The only constant is change."

Understanding what our bodies are going through and how to fully embrace this change while relieving its negative effects can bring you the knowledge and empowerment you need to not only live well, but to thrive.

The truth is, most of the women who are going through menopause aren't talking about it. Instead, they suffer alone with the shame of their symptoms, fighting to just make it through the days as "normally" as possible (normal being how they felt before all these changes started happening).

You are going through "the change." This change is inevitable. You are in perimenopause, or possibly well into menopause, and sometimes when we get here, we just don't recognize ourselves.

The more we learn about menopause, share our own stories, and hear what others are going through, the more we normalize the conversation and bring the truth about ourselves into the light.

This workbook is a conversation starter. A companion for your journey through menopause. A guide and resource to use for yourself or to share with others along your path.

You will find inspiring tips, valuable information, and exercises to add ease to your journey. We've also included fun, uplifting activities and perspectives on every aspect of menopause to "empower yourself to beat the hormone groan!"

Welcome to your adventure of self-discovery:

May you be empowered to beat the Hormone Groan and escape the chains of the Hormone Hostage.

Rate Your Perimenopause Symptoms

During perimenopause and up until menopause, the ovaries are gradually shutting down, making less of the hormones estrogen and progesterone. Hormonal levels can be highly erratic, exhibiting differing fluctuation patterns from month to month, even hour to hour.

The changing levels of these hormones are what trigger perimenopausal symptoms.

Welcome to the Hormone Zone

We have prepared a handy chart to help you rate your hormone symptoms and choose the best martini!

How to Use Your Hormone Symptom Chart

Fill in a Hormone Symptom Chart for three consecutive months. This will reveal patterns and help you notice your symptoms with more clarity.

Follow the scoring instructions below to determine your monthly totals.

Notice your overall pattern of hormone symptoms.

When you become AWARE of your changing hormone symptoms, you are empowered to make changes and adjust your self-care routines before things get out of control.

Score Yourself

If your hormone symptoms are 0–130, your **KINDLING** is starting to burn.
If your hormone symptoms are 131–260, you are on **FIRE**.
If your hormone symptoms are 261–455, you are a **RAGING INFERNO**.

My Hormone Symptom Chart

This Month (#1 of 3) _____

Today's Date _____

Hormone Symptom	Intensity Rating		
	LOW Score 0-10	**MED** Score 11-20	**HIGH** Score 21-35
Changes in occurrence of your period			
Changes in length of your period			
Lighter or heavier flow			
Hot flashes			
Night sweats			
Mood swings			
Mental fog			
Changes in sexual desire			
Bone loss			
Depression and sadness			
Extreme irritability			
Strong food cravings			
Discomfort in the mouth			
My Totals for Month #1:			

TOTAL POINTS: _____ (add all three columns together)

My Hormone Heat Level is (circle one):

KINDLING   FIRE   RAGING INFERNO

My Hormone Symptom Chart

| This Month (#2 of 3) | _____ |
| Today's Date | _____ |

Hormone Symptom	Intensity Rating		
	LOW Score 0-10	**MED** Score 11-20	**HIGH** Score 21-35
Changes in occurrence of your period			
Changes in length of your period			
Lighter or heavier flow			
Hot flashes			
Night sweats			
Mood swings			
Mental fog			
Changes in sexual desire			
Bone loss			
Depression and sadness			
Extreme irritability			
Strong food cravings			
Discomfort in the mouth			
My Totals for Month #2:			

TOTAL POINTS: _____ (add all three columns together)

My Hormone Heat Level is (circle one):

KINDLING   FIRE   RAGING INFERNO

My Hormone Symptom Chart

This Month (#3 of 3) _____

Today's Date _____

Hormone Symptom	Intensity Rating		
	LOW Score 0-10	**MED** Score 11-20	**HIGH** Score 21-35
Changes in occurrence of your period			
Changes in length of your period			
Lighter or heavier flow			
Hot flashes			
Night sweats			
Mood swings			
Mental fog			
Changes in sexual desire			
Bone loss			
Depression and sadness			
Extreme irritability			
Strong food cravings			
Discomfort in the mouth			
My Totals for Month #3:			

TOTAL POINTS: _____ (add all three columns together)

My Hormone Heat Level is (circle one):

KINDLING   FIRE   RAGING INFERNO

Every Woman Is Different

Your journey through menopause will be yours and yours alone. Your story, your experience of the symptoms, and certainly your martini preferences are unique to YOU. This is a time of deep introspection.

No matter what, above everything, you are expressing your own special version of what menopause looks and feels like to YOU.

We hope this workbook gives you tools and ideas to feel empowered on your journey.

We hope that understanding the nuances of each woman's story and understanding there is no good/bad or right/wrong for experiencing menopause in any particular way will open up your journey with more ease and peace.

Here are a couple of mantras for owning your unique position in the parade of women going through menopause:

> **"My unique hormone zone is mine, all mine!"**
>
> **"I am a rock star on my very own hormone stage, singing my very own hit SONG!"**

Martini to the Rescue

Try each of our Top 3 Favorite
Martini/Mocktini recipes
to cool your heat level

#1 If your Hormone Heat Level is KINDLING, try the Party Hearty Martini.

Party Hearty Martini Recipe (found on p. 40 of the book)

- 2 oz vodka
- ½ oz violet liquor
- ½ oz cranberry juice
- splash of soda water
- cake decorating sprinkles

1. Rim top of glass with cranberry juice.
2. Tip upside down into a plate of cake sprinkles.
3. Shake alcohols and juice vigorously, pour into party glass.
4. Top with soda.

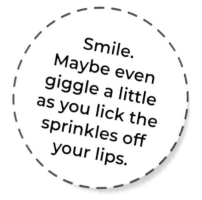

Smile. Maybe even giggle a little as you lick the sprinkles off your lips.

Party Hearty Mocktini Recipe

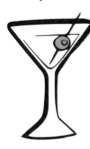

- 2 oz soda water or lemon-lime soda
- ½ oz violet flavoring
- ½ oz cranberry juice
- cake decorating sprinkles

1. Rim top of glass with cranberry juice.
2. Tip upside down into a plate of cake sprinkles.
3. Pour cranberry juice and soda into a shaker with ice, stir, strain, and pour into party glass.

#2 If your Hormone Heat Level is FIRE, try the Artic Cool Martini.

Arctic Cool Martini Recipe (found on p. 83 in the book)

- 2 oz soda water
- ½ oz crème de menthe
- 2 slices fresh lemon
- fresh basil
- fresh mint

1. Muddle basil, mint, and lemon together.
2. Add vodka and crème de menthe.
3. Shake vigorously together with ice and strain.
4. Pour into chilled martini glass.
5. Garnish with fresh basil and mint leaves.

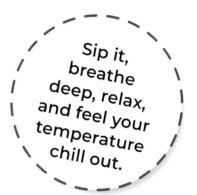

Sip it, breathe deep, relax, and feel your temperature chill out.

Arctic Cool Mocktini Recipe

- 4 oz soda water
- 4 oz mint tea
- 2 slices fresh lemon
- honey to taste
- fresh basil
- fresh mint

1. Muddle basil, mint, and two slices of lemon together.
2. Steep two mint tea bags in 8 ounces of hot water for 5 minutes. Discard tea bags.
3. Add half of tea and a few drops of honey to muddled ingredients.
4. Vigorously shake together with ice, strain.
5. Pour into chilled martini glass.
6. Top with soda.
7. Garnish with fresh mint and basil leaves.

#3 If your Hormone Heat Level is RAGING INFERNO, try The Screamin' O Martini.

The Screamin' O Martini Recipe (found on p. 141 in the book)

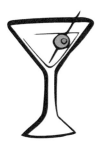

- 2 ½ oz vodka
- 1 oz coconut water
- ½ oz simple syrup
- 3 Amarena cherries
- lemon-lime soda
- half-n-half

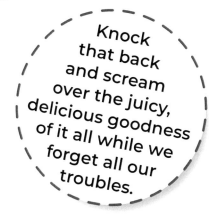

Knock that back and scream over the juicy, delicious goodness of it all while we forget all our troubles.

1. Muddle two Amarena cherries with a teaspoon of its syrup.
2. Add vodka, coconut water, and simple syrup. Shake thoroughly.
3. Pour into chilled martini glass.
4. Top with lemon-lime soda and a splash of half-n-half.
5. Garnish with a cherry.

The Screamin' O Mocktini Recipe

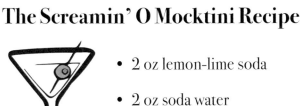

- 2 oz lemon-lime soda
- 2 oz soda water
- 2 oz coconut water
- 3 Amarena cherries
- half-n-half

1. Muddle two Amarena cherries with a teaspoon of its syrup.
2. Add sodas and coconut water. Stir.
3. Pour into chilled martini glass.
4. Add a splash of half-n-half. Garnish with a cherry.

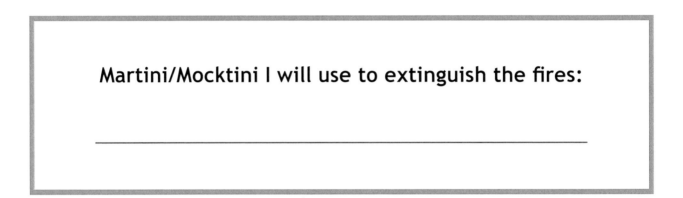

Martini/Mocktini I will use to extinguish the fires:

_____

Chapter One
Brain Fog

WHAT DID I COME
IN HERE FOR...?

Can you relate to Aimee,
who identifies with her sharp
intellect yet finds herself mentally
floundering in a soupy fog?

Loss of focus or short-term memory can be a very real menopausal symptom.

Let's explore your experience with the challenges of feeling forgetful, not being able to remember the way you used to, not having the quick responses you took for granted.

Self-Reflection

Describe a period of brain fog you experienced. What did you forget? What happened?

_____

_____

_____

_____

Was there a negative consequence to this episode? How did that make you feel?

_____

_____

_____

_____

Strategies and Action Steps

Refer to the Take Action section in the book at the end of Chapter 1. The complete list of suggestions and details will help you use the power of ACTION to move from brain fog into brain sunshine!

Highlight your favorite strategy from the book and write it in your own words as if you are making a commitment to yourself.

_____

_____

_____

_____

Make a Five Senses Happiness List.

What sights, sounds, smells, tastes, and touches bring you pleasure?

_____

_____

_____

_____

_____

Get yourself out there!

What will you do this week to network with others?

_____

_____

_____

_____

_____

Dream a little.

What is something new you would like to do or try in the next three months?

_____

_____

_____

_____

_____

Additional Notes:

Additional Notes:

Chapter Two
The Bitch

Can you relate to Christine, who feels so overwhelmed with her body's changes that irritability and impatience have her behaving like a "bitch"?

Hormone-driven "bitchiness" can be a very real menopausal symptom.

Focusing your mind on healing thoughts and intentional self-awareness will help you in times where you are triggered. Our fluctuating hormones cause us to feel bitchy in ways we've never felt before. Self-care to the rescue!

Self-Reflection

Describe a situation when you felt irritated with someone else or found yourself unleashing your bitchy side.

_____

_____

_____

_____

What are the triggers that influence your own irritability—or bitchiness?

_____

_____

_____

Strategies and Action Steps

Refer to the Take Action section in the book at the end of Chapter 2. The complete list of suggestions and details will help you use the power of ACTION to move from bitchy self into lovely self!

Highlight your favorite strategy from the book and write it in your own words as if you are making a commitment to yourself.

_____

_____

_____

Take inventory of what's in those cupboards.

Make a plan for eating. Throw away the processed foods, and replace them with organic, whole foods.

_____

_____

_____

_____

_____

Check your self-talk.

For two days, pay attention to the kinds of messages you allow to run through your brain.

_____

_____

_____

_____

_____

Revisit your Five-Senses Happiness List.

List what's working, what's not working, and what you want to change.

_____

_____

_____

_____

_____

Additional Notes:

Additional Notes:

Games Are Good for the Brain

"Play is our brain's
favorite way of learning."

– Diane Ackerman

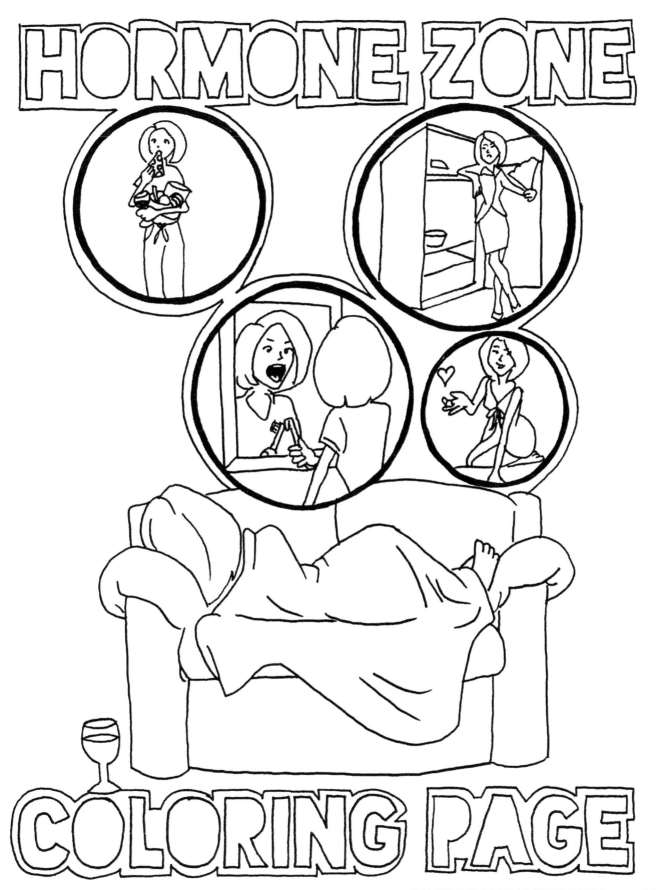

Chapter Three
Basement Blues

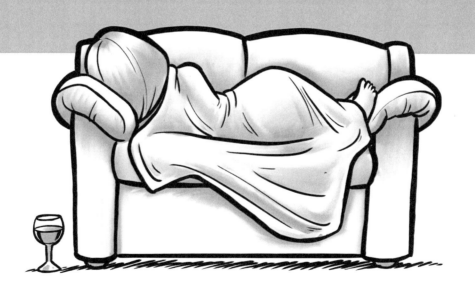

Can you relate to Elaine, who
doesn't want to get out of bed?

Hormone-driven depression can be a very real menopausal symptom.

Let's get in touch with your depressed feelings related to the changes in your body and mind. Do you notice more sad feelings? Do you feel like you can't shake the blues, or you're stuck in a struggle, or you're just perpetually bummed about everything that's going on with you?

Self-Reflection

Describe what it feels like when you are depressed. What do you notice in your body or your thoughts when you feel down, sad, or stuck?

_____

_____

_____

_____

How do you see the connection between your experience of "basement blues" and your hormones?

_____

_____

_____

_____

A Meditation to Lift Your Mood:

Bring to mind the image of a beautiful sunny realm surrounded by a stormy cloud cover. Just like the weather, this cloud cover moves away to reveal the sunshine. With each breath, imagine the cloud cover leaving and settling into the truth that the sunny realm is always there, always available for you to access.

Strategies and Action Steps

Refer to the Take Action section in the book at the end of Chapter 3. The complete list of suggestions and details will help you use the power of ACTION to move from the blues to the rainbows!

Highlight your favorite strategy from the book and write it in your own words as if you are making a commitment to yourself.

_____

_____

_____

_____

Get moving.
List three activities you will use to get up out of bed, get moving, and boost your energy when you feel low on mood and energy.

_____

_____

_____

_____

Pick three positive affirmations for yourself—make them personal.
Write them down, and at least once a day say them out loud.

_____

_____

_____

_____

Hang out with someone who really likes you and sees your value.
Ask them what they like about you. Ask them what your top three strengths or favorite qualities are and write them down. Review them often to lift your spirits.

_____

_____

_____

_____

Additional Notes:

Chapter Four
Periods Unleashed

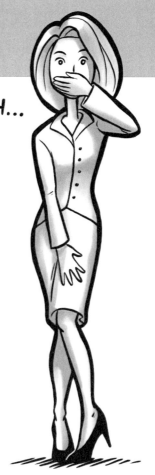

UH OH...

Can you relate to Helen, who is a proud, confident, highly sexual woman just starting to experience frustrating, fluctuating periods?

Hormonal changes interrupting normal period cycles can be a very real menopausal symptom.

Let's investigate how your fluctuating periods affect your ability to know how to prepare for "Aunt Flo" the way you used to. Let's also look at how your changing body can still be sensual and deserves to be adored.

Self-Reflection

Describe what you are experiencing with your changing periods and how it's affecting your life (physically AND emotionally).

_____

_____

_____

_____

What are your favorite ways to express your sensual side? How can you do this regardless of your changing flow?

_____

_____

_____

A Meditation to Hold Your Center:

Imagine feeling grounded in your own changing flow, as if you are happily floating down a river in a safe and sturdy boat. This beautiful river has changing scenery and new currents as you round each bend in the landscape. You are calm, happy, and safe.

Strategies and Action Steps

Refer to the Take Action section in the book at the end of Chapter 4. The complete list of suggestions and details will help you use the power of ACTION to move from frustrated to fabulous!

Highlight your favorite strategy from the book and write it in your own words as if you are making a commitment to yourself.

_____

_____

_____

_____

If you are still having periods, start keeping track.
Write down the day you start, how long you flow, and what the flow is like.

_____

_____

_____

_____

Put together your own menstrual emergency kit.
Always be prepared for the unexpected. What is in your kit?

_____

_____

_____

_____

Discuss with your medical provider.
What are the best options for managing your periods during this transitional phase?

_____

_____

_____

_____

Additional Notes:

Games Are Good for the Brain

"Play is not frivolous; it's not a luxury. Play is important. Play is a drive, a need, a brain-building must-do."

– Jeff A. Johnson

Beat the Hormone Groan Crossword Puzzle

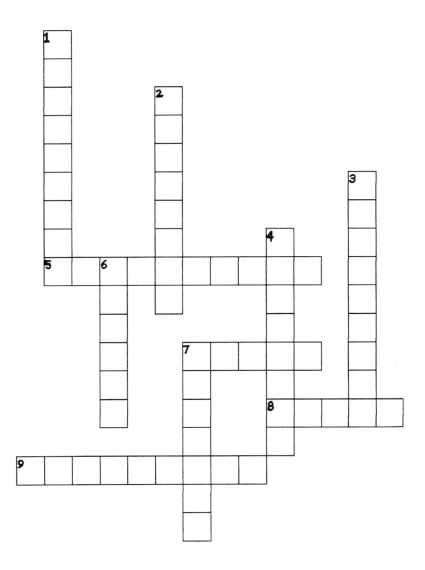

ACROSS

5. Feeling the "basement blues"
7. Goes from regular to irregular
8. 7–9 hours, PLEASE!
9. Feelings all over the map

DOWN

1. The reason for using this workbook
2. The ingredients of menopause
3. A better word than "bitchy"
4. Also known as a "power surge"
6. Here one month, gone the next
7. Give me chips, chocolate, ANYTHING!

ANSWERS: 1-Down: Empowered, 2-Down: Hormones, 3-Down: Irritable, 4-Down: Hot flash, 5-Across: Depression, 6-Down: Period, 7-Down: Craving, 7-Across: Cycle, 8-Across: Sleep, 9-Across: Mood swing

Chapter Five
The Hot Flash

Can you relate to Jennifer, who is efficient and works hard to get it ALL done— but is now facing hot flashes blocking her sense of "being in control"?

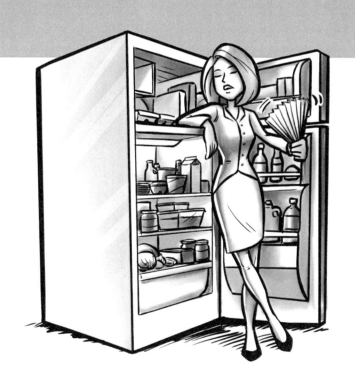

Changes in hormone levels causing intense reactions in the body's physiology can be a very real menopausal symptom.

Let's expand awareness around your feelings of not being in charge, not being able to stay on track, or not having the energy or focus.

Self-Reflection

Write about your top three "hot flash moments," including your thoughts and feelings about them.

_____

_____

_____

_____

Describe your hot flashes as if they have a beginning, a middle, and an end.

_____

_____

_____

_____

Strategies and Action Steps

Refer to the Take Action section in the book at the end of Chapter 5. The complete list of suggestions and details will help you use the power of ACTION to move from out of control to in charge!

Highlight your favorite strategy from the book and write it in your own words as if you are making a commitment to yourself.

_____

_____

_____

_____

Make a plan for exercise.

Find a friend to exercise with. Write down your plan. Do it.

_____

_____

_____

_____

Pick one or two foods high in phytoestrogens. (Refer to Chapter 5 in the book for information on phytoestrogens.)

Eat and/or cook with them for 1–2 weeks.

_____

_____

_____

_____

Go shopping for something new to wear.

Choose items that will wick sweat away and make you feel good! Make a shopping list here. Find an outfit to celebrate your success in the Hormone Zone.

_____

_____

_____

_____

Additional Notes:

Additional Notes:

Chapter Six
Night Sweats

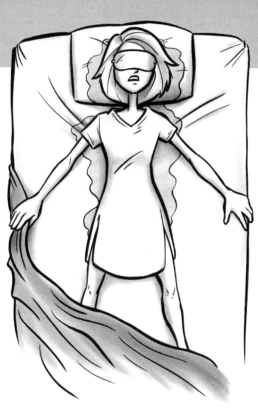

Can you relate to Nadine, who feels like she is "walking through mud" from sleepless nights due to uncontrollable sweating?

Hormonal changes that cause the body to sweat can be a very real menopausal symptom.

Let's get in touch with your feelings about waking up in a sweat at night. How is interrupted sleep affecting your moods and energy? Are you struggling with feeling tired and depleted after nights of waking up multiple times soaked in sweat?

Self-Reflection

Describe what goes through your mind when you are lying in sweaty sheets at night. No editing, just let everything out.

_____

_____

_____

_____

What do you believe are triggers for your night sweats (physical AND emotional)?

_____

_____

_____

_____

Strategies and Action Steps

Refer to the Take Action section in the book at the end of Chapter 6. The complete list of suggestions and details will help you use the power of ACTION to move from sweaty to sweetness!

Highlight your favorite strategy from the book and write it in your own words as if you are making a commitment to yourself.

_____

_____

_____

Practice deep, slow breathing, in and out, three times.

Breathe in to the count of five, hold your breath for five seconds, slowly breathe out for five seconds. Do this at least two times daily and as you lay down to sleep. Track how many times you do this every day and every week. How does deep breathing make you feel?

_____

_____

_____

_____

Identify your personal triggers by keeping a log for one week.

In the morning, after having night sweats, think back to the evening before—identify emotional and physical things you believe triggered the night sweats.

_____

_____

_____

_____

Purchase bamboo sheets and pillowcases.

Research ways to make your bedroom more comfortable, such as adding fans, keeping soft towels next to your bed, or having items handy that help you relax, such as lavender or essential oils with relaxing qualities.

Make a list of items you would like to add to your bedroom:

_____

_____

_____

_____

Additional Notes:

Additional Notes:

Games Are Good
for the Brain

"That's what games are in
the end: Teachers. Fun is just
another word for learning."

– Ralph Koster

Word Scramble

Unscramble each of the clue words.

EOHSRNMO   _ _ _ _ _ _ _ _

RIIMANT   _ _ _ _ _ _ _

NEMPOUSAE   _ _ _ _ _ _ _ _ _

TOH   LSAFH   _ _ _   _ _ _ _ _

TIGHN   WEASST   _ _ _ _ _   _ _ _ _ _ _

MDOO   WINSSG   _ _ _ _   _ _ _ _ _ _

FODO   CANVSGIR   _ _ _ _   _ _ _ _ _ _ _ _

RIILABTIIRYT   _ _ _ _ _ _ _ _ _ _ _ _

AKCB   TAF   _ _ _ _   _ _ _

EENOISPSDR   _ _ _ _ _ _ _ _ _ _

Chapter Seven

I Want My Wine & Chips!

Can you relate to Toby, who has always been a healthy eater yet feels like she's on a self-loathing rollercoaster of weird food cravings that have her eating greasy chips at night?

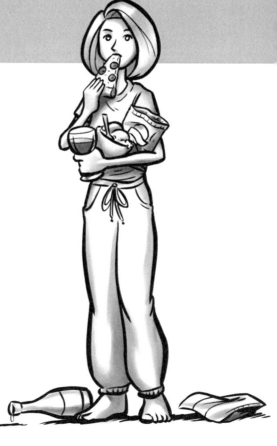

Hormonal changes that cause food cravings can be a very real menopausal symptom.

Let's explore your out-of-control snacking, chowing down, or pigging out. Do you feel like your food cravings are stronger and your willpower to say no to binge eating is lower than ever?

Self-Reflection

Describe your experiences with food cravings and your attempts to satisfy them, whether successful or unsuccessful. Share in full.

_____

_____

_____

_____

Recall a time when you felt strong and "on top of your game" with food choices.

_____

_____

_____

_____

A Meditation for Self-Forgiveness

Connect with your compassion, letting it fill your heart
as you begin breathing long, slow, deep breaths.

Connect with your natural ability to forgive
yourself when you are surrounded by LOVE.
Place all else into the transformative fire
and let only the love remain.

Strategies and Action Steps

Refer to the Take Action section in the book at the end of Chapter 7. The complete list of suggestions and details will help you use the power of ACTION to move from guilt-food-binging to happy-healthy-snacking!

Highlight your favorite strategy from the book and write it in your own words as if you are making a commitment to yourself.

_____

_____

_____

_____

Keep a food diary for one week.
List your food cravings: what specific foods you crave, when you crave them, and what you think triggers the cravings.

_____

_____

_____

_____

Choose two strategies to reduce giving in to your cravings.
Will you take a walk after dinner? Will you call a friend to check in with them?

_____

_____

_____

_____

Choose a reward for meeting your food behavior goal.
Write your desired behavior change and what you will do to earn your reward.

_____

_____

_____

Schedule exercise this week.

Sweat to get your dopamine and serotonin levels up through the roof! Make at least two exercise dates with yourself, and keep them.

_____

_____

_____

_____

Additional Notes:

Chapter Eight
Back Fat & Jelly Rolls

Can you relate to Linda, Carol, and Mona, who each struggle with body-fat changes, leaving them feeling frustrated, obsessed, and critical of their physical appearance?

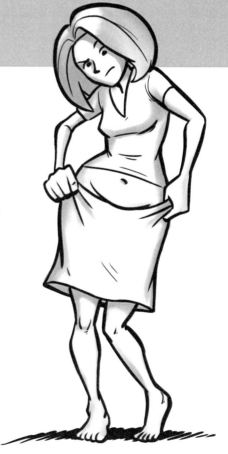

Hormone-driven weight gain can be a very real menopausal symptom.

Let's get in touch with the fear of not being able to lose the weight, of not being able to maintain the way you "used to look," or of not being confident with your physical appearance.

Self-Reflection

Describe what you see happening to your body's appearance at this stage of life.

_____

_____

_____

_____

What are your emotions and attitudes toward your changing body?

_____

_____

_____

_____

Strategies and Action Steps

Refer to the Take Action section in the book at the end of Chapter 8. The complete list of suggestions and details will help you use the power of ACTION to move from flabby to fabulous!

Highlight your favorite strategy from the book and write it in your own words as if you are making a commitment to yourself:

_____

_____

_____

_____

Recharge your Adrenals.

Track your weekly consumption of processed foods and simple sugars. List healthy, whole food alternatives you could replace them with.

_____

_____

_____

_____

Examine your sleep habits.

List five things you can SAY NO to doing in the evenings to support healthy sleep

_____

_____

_____

_____

Exercise. Exercise. Exercise.

Find new ways to move. Make a list of activities you can do that would feel FUN. Ask others what fun exercise choices they make. Try one at a time and build up a personal exercise regimen.

_____

_____

_____

_____

Additional Notes:

Additional Notes:

Games Are Good for the Brain

"We don't stop playing because
we grow old, we grow old
because we stop playing."
– George Bernard Shaw

Self-Love Maze: The Journey into Your Center

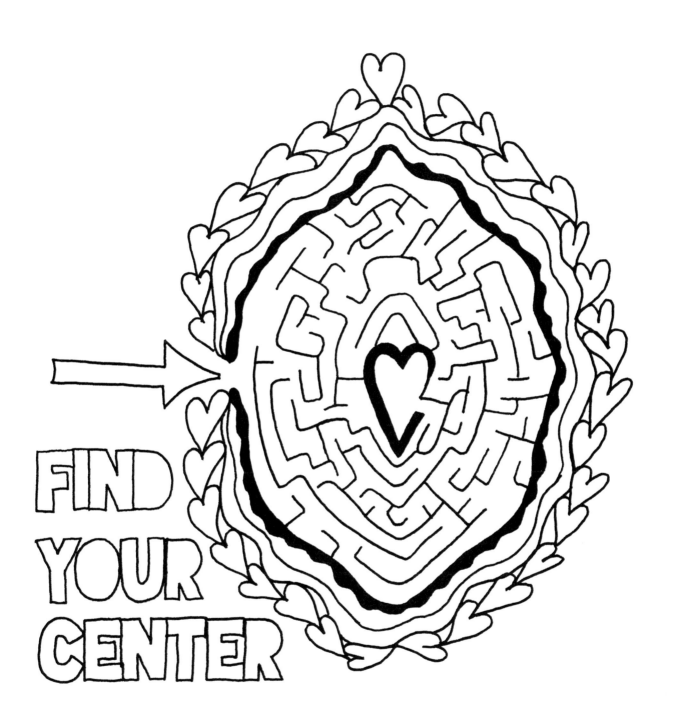

Chapter Nine
Mouth on Fire

Can you relate to Teresa, who is surprised she has to deal with bad breath, teeth, and gum issues at this time in her life?

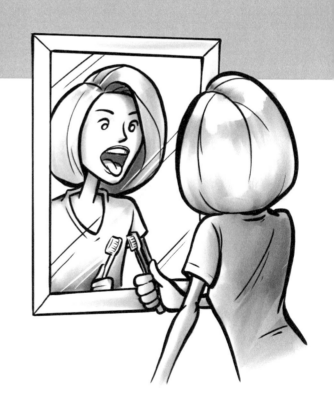

Estrogen levels changing inside the mouth can be a very real menopausal symptom.

Let's explore what feelings come up when facing uncomfortable issues related to your mouth, the way you smile, the lack of confidence in your breath, or worry about your teeth.

Self-Reflection

Describe what it feels like to become aware of your mouth (even if it's positive or negative awareness).

_____

_____

_____

_____

What are your current daily habits that keep your mouth healthy?

_____

_____

_____

_____

Strategies and Action Steps

Refer to the Take Action section in the book at the end of Chapter 9.

> Sometimes, as you age, your body's changes force you to face uncomfortable issues related to the look of your smile or changes in the smell of your breath, and you worry about your teeth like you've never had to before. Let's explore this here.

Highlight your favorite strategy from the book and write it in your own words as if you are making a commitment to yourself:

_____

_____

_____

_____

Make your teeth brushing time MINDFUL.

Practice being present in the moment when you are caring for your teeth. Describe ways you can add mindfulness to the time you spend brushing.

_____

_____

_____

_____

Research toothpaste and mouth rinse ingredients.

Look for SLS-free products if you are having mouth symptoms. List some product options here or products you want to avoid for your own reference. What do you currently use to clean your mouth? Do your products have SLS in them? Check the labels.

_____

_____

_____

_____

Do something every day to relieve your stress.

List your favorites or "go-to choices" for stress relief. Choose your top three things and choose a way you can stay accountable to practice them daily.

_____

_____

_____

_____

Additional Notes:

Chapter Ten
Let's Talk Sex, Baby

Can you relate to Mary, who has loved sex all her life but can't make sense of her inability to orgasm or her decreased sexual desires?

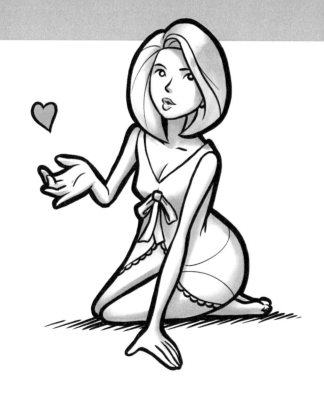

Hormone-driven sexual responses can be a very real menopausal symptom.

Let's put positive energy around your feelings of inadequacy or loss in your sex life. Become aware of feeling different about your orgasm or what has changed around your desires, arousal, or stamina in the bedroom. Notice your judgment or fears about your sexual expression and what it means to feel insecure when it comes to sex.

Self-Reflection

Describe a situation when you felt awkward about sex or your own sexuality.

_____

_____

_____

_____

If this is an opportunity for you to re-invent your sexual self and you are completely fearless, what would it look like?

_____

_____

_____

_____

Strategies and Action Steps

Refer to the Take Action section in the book at the end of Chapter 10. The complete list of suggestions and details will help you use the power of ACTION to move from struggling to sexy!

Highlight your favorite strategy from the book and write it in your own words as if you are making a commitment to yourself.

_____

_____

_____

Make your own list of feel-good, exciting sexual activities.

Include things to inspire your imagination when it comes to feeling sexual. Include fun activities that motivate your sexy side.

_____

_____

_____

_____

_____

See a women's health specialist.

Explore hormone therapy, hormone vaginal supplements, or other treatments to help you get back that lovin' feeling. List your options.

_____

_____

_____

_____

_____

Additional Notes:

Additional Notes:

The Fantastic 4

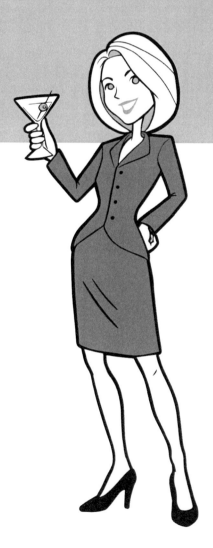

In my research and writing for the book *Martinis & Menopause*, four areas consistently came up regarding how to eliminate or reduce many of the symptoms women face during the menopausal transition.

I call these the Fantastic4.

Living as our best selves means we feel good mentally and physically. Even through the ups and downs of shifting hormones and the differing circumstances of our lives, we can make small, doable changes to our daily routines.

This workbook is your companion to make the Fantastic4 work for you:

1. **Exercise**
2. **Food Choices**
3. **Hormone Replacement Therapy**
4. **Sleep**

The Fantastic4 will catapult you out of the Hormone Hostage Zone and into the wonderful space of living better and feeling better.

Disclaimer: I am not an exercise science major, a nutritionist, or a doctor. But I do know things that work—to keep us living better and free us from being a Hormone Hostage!

My Fantastic4 Empowering Choices

Wherever you are in your menopausal journey—just starting, in the midst of it all, or post—creating your own choices will help you live your best self.

If you commit to working on these four areas, picking a couple of things you can adjust or modify, you will have the power to change your life and to escape the Hormone Hostage Zone.

Write your most empowering choice in each Fantastic4 area.

My Exercise Choice:

_____

_____

_____

_____

My Food Choice:

_____

_____

_____

_____

My Hormone Replacement Choice:

_____

_____

_____

_____

My Sleep Hygiene Choice:

_____

_____

_____

_____

Fantastic4 Exercise Choices

Activity: Your 15-Minute Dance Party

Exercise is the first line of defense to breaking free from the Hormone Hostage Zone.

Vigorous exercise has been stressed throughout the book for its almost magical properties (pp. 155–156). Magical because the benefits of getting your sexy sweat on are immense and positively affect nearly every menopausal symptom and bodily system.

The North American Menopause Society—the leading voice of menopause—states the following:

> Exercise may cause the same magnitude of
> change as that induced by estrogen therapy.

15-Minute Dance Party Instructions:

Let's make exercising simple and fun.

Do you love to move or dance? Put your favorite type of music on and let yourself loose for at least 15 minutes. If the average song is 3 minutes, give yourself 5 songs, and you have reached your daily goal of for cardio/movement.

Let the music help you get your heart rate up! And work up into a sweat!

Activity: What's on My Motivation Board?

Vision boards are great for motivating yourself to reach goals. Let's make a Motivation Board to keep yourself on track with your exercise choices. Use this collection of images to remind your fun-loving brain that positive energy comes from exercise and you are ready and willing to participate fully. Whether you love to exercise or don't like it at all, we can agree that it's your number one strategy to navigate menopause successfully.

Collect several images that inspire you around the following statements:

I love to move.

I love feeling energized.

I love the feeling of strength in my body.

My mood lifts when my body is moving.

Dancing lifts my spirits and my energy.

Glue the images on any size poster board.

Keep it simple. Even two or three images on a small card will do the job!

Ignite your positive feelings, and your
exercise goals will be easier to reach.

Fantastic4 Food Choices

Activity: What's in My Cupboard?

It's important to set yourself up for success by filling your kitchen with ingredients for cooking healthy "menopause-supportive" meals. The more you can prepare foods to eat on the go, or to have handy at home, the easier it will be to overcome the hormone groan.

Based on the book, list the top ten items you choose to have in your kitchen for eating and cooking.

My Menopause-Supportive Cupboard

1. _____
2. _____
3. _____
4. _____
5. _____
6. _____
7. _____
8. _____
9. _____
10. _____

Omega3 Rich Foods: (Be sure to include these):

- Flax seeds, chia seeds, and their oils
- Seafood, especially fatty fish like salmon, tuna, mackerel, halibut, trout, oyster
- Nuts, especially walnuts
- Soybeans
- Vegetable oils, like olive and coconut
- Green leafy vegetables, like spinach, kale, and broccoli
- Dietary supplements containing omega3
- Whole grains

Activity: My Favorite Menopause Meals

Create a meal or snack using your Menopause-Supportive Cupboard.

MEAL/SNACK #1:

Veggie _____

Protein _____

Healthy Fat _____

MEAL/SNACK #2:

Veggie _____

Protein _____

Healthy Fat _____

MEAL/SNACK #3:

Veggie _____

Protein _____

Healthy Fat _____

> Remember, meals high in organic vegetables and lean organic protein, whole grains, and healthy fats are essential to helping menopausal women look and feel better.

Resources:

- www.everydayhealth.com/hs/guide-to-managing-menopause/the-optimal-menopause-diet/
- www.webmd.com/menopause/guide/staying-healthy-through-good-nuitrition#1

Fantastic4 HRT Choices

Become a Detective

Hormone Replacement Therapy (HRT) has been shown to improve the life of menopausal women, helping with hot flashes, bone and brain health, and emotional stability.

Starting HRT earlier in the menopausal transition—rather than later—has a positive effect on your changing body.

NOTE: *Unless you are at risk for estrogen-fed cancers, HRT can be explored.*

> Like Sherlock Holmes sleuthing out a mystery, be a detective and find out who treats women with HRT in your area.

Investigate the following sources (BESIDES your primary care doctor):
- Naturopath
- Chiropractor
- Nurse Practitioner
- OB/GYN or Women's Health Clinic

How to Find Clues:
1. Locate the pharmacy in your area that offers bio-identical hormones. Call them and ask for the practitioner information of who is prescribing HRT. Ask who uses their pharmacy to fulfill scripts.
2. Check out the North American Menopause Society website to search for practitioners in your area (www.menopause.org/for-women/find-a-menopause-practitioner.)
3. Sleuth out providers at Bio-T Medical (www.biotemedical.com/bioidentical-hormone-replacement-therapy-provider.)

My HRT Discovery Log

Medical Providers or Holistic Practitioners who provide HRT and support for menopausal woman

Name	Location	Phone/Email
1.		
2.		
3.		
4.		
5.		
6.		
7.		
8.		
9.		
10.		

My Detective Notes: Information from Pharmacies

Who	Where	Contact
1.		
2.		
3.		
4.		
5.		
6.		
7.		
8.		
9.		
10.		

Activity: Serve Yourself!

Self-care goes a long way to add ease and success to your hormonal experiences during menopause. HRT can be extremely helpful, especially when you make educated decisions that are in your own PERSONAL best interest.

Practice self-care by choosing how you want to "serve yourself the very best!"

Delivery Methods for HRT
- Transdermal: Under the Skin
- Pellets
- Creams
- Vaginal Suppositories
- Lozenges
- Under the Tongue
- Patches

Investigate your own preferences to make the best choices.
Which method fits best into your daily routine and lifestyle?

_____

_____

Which method would make it easy and effortless?

_____

_____

Which method do you need more information to understand better?

_____

_____

Which method would you NOT want to use?

_____

_____

Describe the "HRT of your dreams" and what steps you need to take to make these dreams a reality for you.

_____

_____

_____

_____

_____

_____

_____

_____

_____

_____

_____

_____

_____

_____

_____

_____

Fantastic4 Sleep Choices

Activity: My Nightly Sleep Hygiene Routine

Issues surrounding sleep have hit the mainstream. Thankfully, there are many resources and healthy sleep tips now available online that are easy to access.

The term "sleep hygiene" implies a cool and hip context where improvement is made easy and fun.

> Definition: Sleep hygiene is a variety of different practices that are necessary to have normal, quality nighttime sleep and full daytime alertness.

Example of a Sleep-Ready Routine:

I stop all electronics at least thirty minutes before bed. I stop drinking alcohol at least one hour before bed. I drink a big glass of water. I stop answering my phone. I stop eating. I take my nighttime supplements (progesterone and melatonin). I wash my face and brush my teeth. I apply a deliciously scented lotion to my skin. I turn off all lights in my bedroom except the lamp by my bedside. Once in bed, I breathe deeply, close my eyes, and play back my day. Anything that was unpleasant or particularly stressful, I mentally breathe out and let go of. I then think about the good parts of the day, and I make a mental list of all that I am grateful for. After that, I turn my mind to tomorrow and imagine the day in my head, what I will do, and what successes I will have, putting a positive vibe out into the universe about tomorrow. I pick up my book and read until ready for sleep.

Create Your Own "Getting Ready for Sleep" Routine.

Make sure it speaks to your heart and feels realistic.

_____

_____

_____

_____

_____

_____

_____

_____

10 Areas of Positive Sleep Hygiene

Rate yourself in each area to determine where to make changes for the better.

1. Have a "getting ready for sleep routine"   Good ___   Needs Improvement ___

2. Reduce alcohol and heavy meals before bed   Good ___   Needs Improvement ___

3. Make your bedroom a sanctuary   Good ___   Needs Improvement ___

4. Create an environment of darkness for sleeping Good ___   Needs Improvement ___

5. Turn on or see natural light upon waking   Good ___   Needs Improvement ___

6. Eliminate TV or computers in the bedroom   Good ___   Needs Improvement ___

7. Regulate your sleeping hours (consistency)   Good ___   Needs Improvement ___

8. Keep your bedroom cool   Good ___   Needs Improvement ___

9. Wear loose-fitting or no clothes for sleeping Good ___   Needs Improvement ___

10. Try for 7–9 hours of sleep nightly   Good ___   Needs Improvement ___

Activity: Set Goals for Stellar Sleep Hygiene!

Set one simple goal for the following areas of positive sleep hygiene:

Reduce alcohol/heavy meals before bed:

_____

_____

Sleep in darkness:

_____

_____

See natural light upon waking:

_____

_____

No TV or computer in bedroom:

_____

_____

Regular sleeping hours:

_____

_____

Keep bedroom cool:

_____

_____

Comfortable sleepwear:

_____

_____

Get 7–9 hours nightly:

_____

_____

Choose one of the sleep hygiene areas as your FOCUS GOAL to start.

My #1 FOCUS GOAL:

_____

_____

_____

_____

Write down your Action Steps:

_____

_____

_____

_____

_____

_____

_____

_____

_____

_____

_____

_____

_____

_____

_____

_____

My Menopause Mantras

How to create your own Mantra to support your success in each area of the Fantastic4:

(Note: *A mantra is a positive affirmation*)

Step 1: Fill in the blanks.

A menopause symptom I struggle with:

_____

_____

Why this symptom is challenging:

_____

_____

My #1 negative thought about this symptom/challenge:

_____

_____

Step 2: Rewrite each answer into a positive statement.

My (write your symptom) _____ is/are my superpower.

Rewrite the challenge into an opportunity:

_____

_____

Rewrite the negative thought into a positive one:

_____

_____

_____

EXAMPLE: Answers to Step #1

I struggle with hot flashes.

Hot flashes are challenging because they distract me, and it's already become harder and harder to focus these days.

I'm embarrassed to have hot flashes, and they make me feel inadequate.

EXAMPLE: Positive Mantras Step #2

My hot flashes are my superpower!

The distraction gives me a much needed mini-break, and I can come back into focus gently and easily.

I visualize my hot flashes as a positive source of energy meant to feed my soul if I just allow it.

Now write your own Menopause Mantra:

_____

_____

_____

_____

_____

_____

_____

_____

Meditation for Peaceful Menopause

Suggestion: Record this meditation in your own voice using your smartphone. Play it back to yourself once each day when you can sit quietly with your eyes closed.

Imagine yourself climbing up a lovely mountainside toward a vista point overlooking a huge valley with beautiful wildflowers growing throughout.

Lengthen your breathing and begin telling yourself that you can see and be everything and anything you want JUST AS YOU ARE.

Thank yourself for your changing rhythms.

Feel gratitude for the movement and change within.

Anticipate with a peaceful heart your new pace on all levels: mind, body, and spirit.

Imagine you are seeing this valley in slow motion—able to soak up every beautiful detail. Give yourself permission to personalize your own view of what's before you.

Imagine every colorful flower as a nugget of the changing YOU.

Imagine you are a bouquet of wildflowers, fresh and new and inspiring.

As you exhale, leave behind any negative belief about your changing hormones and breathe it out into the nourishing valley floor.

Take your time to transition from your internal world back out to the external world by placing your bouquet of wildflowers into your heart to keep with you.

About the Author

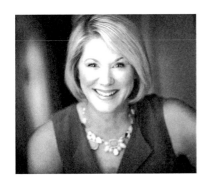

Kelli Jaecks is a prolific speaker, blogger, and lover of life!

Her book *Martinis & Menopause* was inspired by her own journey through menopause and her passion for helping women feel better and live better.

When not speaking or writing, Kelli enjoys performing in live theater and traveling to cool venues for scuba diving. She lives in Oregon with her husband.

What is a Martinis & Menopause Soirée?

Let's Soirée! Kelli Jaecks may soon be coming to your town!

A soirée is a social event held in private homes or at local businesses in cities across the United States that combine a cocktail party atmosphere with valuable, practical information.

These fun, educational, women-celebrated events create a setting that encourages open dialogue on women's health and wellness issues focused on perimenopause, menopause, and postmenopausal issues.

Contact Kelli to schedule an appearance.

Kelli is available to visit your soirée, book club, group, or event either in-person or through video conference. She loves talking to groups about her personal journey through menopause, her writing process, and facilitating inspiring conversations with her readers.

www.kellijaecks.com   kelli@kellijaecks.com   503-881-5633

Follow Kelli on social media:
@kellijaecks   @kellijaecksverbalimpact